CONTENTS

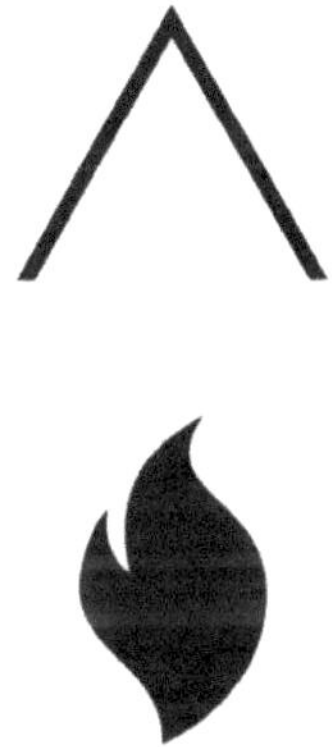

#GawdBowdy

INTRODUCTION

Embarking on a fitness journey is often more challenging than it seems. Achieving meaningful results goes beyond simply lifting weights or following a calisthenics routine. *The Psychology of Working Out* delves into the mental and emotional aspects of exercise, exploring how fitness can elevate confidence, improve health, and enhance overall quality of life.

Success in fitness requires more than physical effort—it demands the right mindset. This guide will help you cultivate that mindset, perfect your techniques for optimal results, and design a workout plan tailored to your unique needs and lifestyle. Whether you're balancing a demanding work schedule or looking for ways to stay motivated, this book provides the tools and insights to help you thrive.

As you read, reflect on the principles shared and put them into practice. This isn't just a guide—it's a roadmap to transformation. By the end of this journey, you'll not only see a change in your physical appearance but also in your mental resilience and personal growth.

Turning the pages of this guide marks the start of a new chapter in your life—one that defines your character as strong, determined, and possibly even legendary. Congratulations on taking the first step toward your goal. Your commitment to self-improvement is already a victory, and I'm proud of you for beginning this journey. Let's get started. Together, we'll turn this resolution into a revolution.

CHAPTER ONE: THE BENEFITS OF WORKING OUT

The benefits of working out are vast and transformative, touching every aspect of your life. While this guide can't cover every advantage, we'll focus on those most profoundly supported by empirical evidence. These benefits are more than just theoretical; they're real, measurable, and life-changing.

Emotional Wellness and Self-Esteem

One of the most significant benefits of working out lies in its impact on emotional health. Your emotional state dictates how you navigate your days, interact with others, and achieve success. It also plays a pivotal role in shaping your self-esteem, which precedes you in all aspects of life. Whether you're pursuing a career, building relationships, or simply walking into a room, your self-esteem signals to others who you are: a confident, capable individual who adds value or someone who struggles with self-doubt.

When you commit to regular exercise, you're making an investment in your emotional well-being. Consider this: starting a workout regimen offers two possible outcomes.

1. **Giving Up**: If you start and quit before reaching your goals, you risk damaging your self-esteem. This sense of failure can erode your emotional state, leaving you

disappointed in yourself.

2. **Seeing It Through**: On the other hand, staying consistent and focusing on your goals fosters immense personal growth. Achieving small victories triggers the release of dopamine, a feel-good chemical that reinforces positive behavior. Over time, this builds confidence and a healthier emotional state. You begin to carry yourself with assurance, knowing you can accomplish what you set out to do.

This newfound consistency and self-belief extend beyond fitness. Whether it's developing a habit of daily reading for mental stimulation or taking part in social improvement initiatives, your reliability and confidence will make you stand out as someone worth knowing.

Physical Health and Longevity

The health benefits of working out are undeniable and well-documented. Regular physical activity improves your cardiovascular system by increasing heart rate and promoting healthy blood circulation. This supports your body's biological processes, ensuring efficiency and vitality. Over time, these benefits accumulate, reducing the risk of chronic diseases and extending lifespan.

Another critical but often overlooked benefit is the impact of exercise on sexual health. Maintaining a consistent workout routine has been linked to a healthier libido, a vital aspect of overall well-being. As we age, it's natural for libido to decline, which can lead to relationship challenges. Exercise helps counteract this by boosting energy, stamina, and hormonal balance, ensuring that both you and your partner feel connected and fulfilled.

Enhanced Quality of Life

Finally, one of the most rewarding benefits of working out is its effect on your overall quality of life. Research shows a strong correlation between physical fitness and personal satisfaction. When you feel good about how you look, your confidence radiates into other areas of life.

As your fitness journey progresses, you'll notice changes not just in your body but in your behavior and mindset. Increased focus, discipline, and energy will naturally earn respect from others. You'll smile more, engage in meaningful conversations, and participate in social activities with renewed enthusiasm.

This transformation is rooted in pride—pride in the goals you've achieved and the hard work you've put in. That self-assurance will become a defining trait, evident in every action you take.
Working out isn't just about physical changes—it's a holistic journey that elevates your emotional state, builds unshakable self-esteem, improves your health, and enhances your quality of life. These benefits, and countless others, make regular exercise not just an option but a necessity for a thriving, fulfilling life. Let this chapter serve as your reminder that each workout brings you closer to a stronger, healthier, and more confident version of yourself.

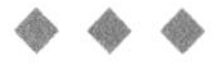

CHAPTER TWO: THE POWER OF MINDSET

Embarking on a journey to transform your body and improve your quality of life begins with the right mindset. Developing this mindset may seem daunting, but it's achievable with the right approach. Your mindset isn't one-size-fits-all; it must align with your unique circumstances and goals.

Consider this analogy: A soldier in wartime needs an alert and focused mindset to be effective in their mission. Similarly, to successfully commit to and maintain a workout routine, you must cultivate a mindset tailored to your fitness journey. And here's a truth you need to embrace early on—this journey is for life.

A Lifelong Commitment

Yes, you read that correctly: working out is a lifetime commitment. While it may sound intimidating, it's a reality for achieving sustained health and fitness. There are no quick fixes or temporary plans that deliver lasting results. Forget the "30-day shred" or "three-month transformation" promises—lasting change requires consistent effort over the long haul.

Before you begin, embrace the idea that fitness isn't a destination but a lifelong journey. This commitment isn't for everyone, but for those who truly desire transformation, it's a mindset worth adopting.

Building Your Mindset

The foundation of a successful workout mindset starts with self-reflection and an honest assessment of your lifestyle. Ask yourself:

- Are you a busy parent struggling to find time for yourself?
- Are you older with limited mobility but determined to improve?
- Are you capable but unmotivated to start a routine?

Regardless of your situation, there's a workout plan that fits your needs. A great starting point for most individuals is three 45-minute sessions per week. This manageable schedule minimizes overwhelm and sets a solid foundation. Once you identify your available time, commit to it. You'll notice an immediate shift in your mindset as you take control of your schedule and prioritize your well-being.

Consistency: The Key Ingredient

Consistency is non-negotiable. It's the bridge between intention and transformation. Anyone can work out occasionally, but the real benefits come from sustained effort. Consistency not only strengthens your body but also reinforces your reputation as a reliable and disciplined individual.

Imagine telling friends and family you're starting a fitness routine, only to quit after a few weeks. This damages your self-esteem and your social credibility. On the other hand, sticking to your commitment inspires respect and trust, both in yourself and from others.

Consistency builds self-confidence and reinforces a positive cycle: completing your workouts releases dopamine, which boosts your mood and encourages further commitment. Over time, this habit will transform how others see you—and how you see yourself.

Focus: Blocking Out Distractions

Focus is another cornerstone of a strong mindset. No matter how dedicated you are, you'll encounter distractions and naysayers along the way. Some people may mock your routine, tempt you with unhealthy habits, or distract you with their own ambitions.

Stay centered. This journey is about *you*. Avoid unnecessary comparisons or competitions with others—they'll only detract from your progress. Genetics, access to resources, and other factors make everyone's fitness journey unique. Focus on your goals and measure success by how far you've come, not by someone else's standards.

Avoid relying on material motivations like gym outfits or supplements to keep you committed. True commitment comes from within, not from external accessories. Similarly, resist the urge to expect immediate recognition or rewards. Success in fitness, as in life, is earned through persistence and humility.

Celebrate Personal Progress

You'll know you're succeeding when the people who matter to you begin to notice your progress without you seeking validation. Their unprompted compliments will reflect the hard work and dedication you've put in. This moment is a powerful affirmation of your growth, both physically and mentally.

Your mindset is the foundation of your fitness journey. By embracing a lifelong commitment, staying consistent, and focusing on your personal growth, you'll set yourself up for success. Remember, this journey is about becoming the best version of yourself. Stay humble, stay focused, and most importantly—stay committed.

Let's move forward, stronger and more determined than ever.

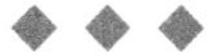

CHAPTER THREE: PSYCHOLOGY

The psychological impact of working out is profound, influencing self-confidence, self-esteem, and behavioral habits. These factors are not only key to fitness but also fundamental to how we navigate life. To truly understand the psychology of working out, we must explore how it transforms your mind as much as your body.

The Role of Self-Confidence

Self-confidence is the invisible force that drives how you walk, talk, and interact with the world. It isn't a rare gift bestowed upon a select few—it's a skill you can develop and refine. Some people command attention the moment they enter a room, while others struggle to be noticed. The difference often lies in confidence.

Working out has a remarkable ability to boost self-confidence. It begins with small, consistent victories. Imagine this scenario: you commit to going to the gym on Monday at 6 PM to work on your upper body. Monday arrives, and you follow through on your plan. This act of planning, executing, and achieving is a direct manifestation of your intentions.

You're not just lifting weights; you're proving to yourself that you can set a goal and accomplish it. That sense of achievement fuels your confidence. Over time, you look better, feel better, and carry yourself with an undeniable assurance. This is the essence of self-confidence—built one small success at a time.

Understanding Self-Esteem

While self-confidence shines outwardly in social situations, self-esteem reflects your inner world. It's how you see yourself when no one else is watching. High self-esteem means you validate your worth from within, not through external approval.

In many ways, self-esteem is the catalyst for self-confidence. When you consistently show up for your workouts, you validate yourself. You said you'd do something, and you did it. This consistency reinforces your belief in your capabilities.

Every rep and every set becomes an investment in your well-being. You're not just sculpting your body; you're building emotional wealth. You become your own source of validation, granting yourself permission to feel happy, accomplished, and deserving of success. Self-esteem becomes the foundation for your confidence and resilience.
Through this lens, your workout routine is much more than a New Year's resolution. It's a transformative journey that strengthens you mentally, physically, and spiritually.

Behavioral Transformation

As you settle into a consistent workout routine, you'll notice subtle but powerful changes in your behavior. The discipline you cultivate in the gym begins to ripple through other areas of your life.

For instance, imagine committing to reading one chapter of a book each day to keep your mind sharp. Before developing discipline, you might rationalize skipping a day due to a social event or fatigue. However, once you've embraced consistency through your workouts, this habit extends naturally to other commitments.

Repetition sharpens your ability to follow through. Just as your body instinctively prepares for a workout at the usual time, your mind becomes wired to complete tasks, whether it's reading, pursuing a professional goal, or sticking to personal promises.

This behavioral shift is captured in a popular saying circulating on social media: *"How you do anything is how you do everything."*
The psychology of working out is a transformative force. It builds your self-confidence, fortifies your self-esteem, and reshapes your behavior to create a foundation for success in all areas of life. By committing to your fitness journey, you're not just improving your body—you're redefining your identity.

Keep this truth close: every small step you take is a victory, every commitment you honor is a triumph, and every habit you build paves the way for a better you. The psychology of working out isn't just about fitness; it's about mastering your mind and living a life of purpose.

◆ ◆ ◆

CHAPTER 4: TECHNIQUE

Technique. The following two chapters are the meat of this book—the core of the content. Without these, everything else falls apart. Proper technique is essential in any workout routine. Without it, you might commit to a regular regimen and see little progress, which could lead to frustration, depression, and a decrease in self-confidence. So, learning technique isn't just important, it's vital.

The Importance of Tailoring Your Technique

Everyone is different. To achieve the best results, you need to tailor your technique to fit your body type, your family genetics, and the resources available to you. This is why it's essential to customize your workout routine to match your specific goals. When you understand how to execute proper form, you'll ensure that your time and effort are well spent.

This technique was developed over six years of trial and error, working closely with military professionals. It's a proven method that can help you see results and avoid common pitfalls.

The Squeeze

The first half of this technique is what I call "the squeeze." The squeeze is responsible for body definition—it's what gets you shredded. During a rep, the primary focus should be the muscle you're targeting. For example, if you're doing a bench press, as you lift the bar, you shouldn't feel much strain in your shoulders or upper back. Instead, you should feel most of the tension in your chest.

To do this correctly:
- As you push the bar up, initiate the movement by squeezing your pectoral muscles, as if you were flexing them.
- Only after this initial squeeze should your arms and back assist in the lift.
- Once the bar reaches its peak, hold it there for a second, continuing to squeeze your chest muscles.
- Then, lower the bar back down slowly, maintaining the squeeze throughout the movement.

This method maximizes the tension on the target muscle, which is key for muscle growth and definition.
For a more practical example, let's take dumbbell curls:
- When you curl the dumbbells, start the motion by squeezing your biceps.
- As you curl, your forearms can assist, but the squeeze should remain the focus.
- Pause at the 90-degree angle, holding the squeeze for a second, and then lower the dumbbell back down slowly.

The squeeze is like getting the benefit of two exercises in one motion—maximizing muscle engagement and growth.

Mastering the Squeeze

To master the squeeze, begin by practicing with no weight. Use a broomstick or an empty barbell to perform your workout. Do this for about two weeks. You might be concerned about how others in the gym will view you lifting air, but remember this: you are the only person who needs to understand why you're doing it.

14

In time, people will see the results of your commitment and will be asking for your advice.

This is your journey. Stay focused on your goal. It's not about impressing others, but about achieving personal growth. Focus on the process and the progress you're making.

The Zone

The second part of the technique is what I call "the zone." The zone refers to the maximum tension points during an exercise. There are certain moments in each rep where the tension on the muscle is at its highest, and it's in these moments where maximum gains occur. For example, when performing a bench press, the maximum tension point is when your elbows are bent at about 45 degrees, with your triceps parallel to your upper back. This is the zone. It's the area where the muscle is under constant tension and working hardest.

When lifting a weight, staying in the zone is crucial for strength training and muscle endurance. By maintaining tension in the zone, you challenge your muscles to perform at their best, ultimately increasing both muscle definition and strength.

Practicing the Zone

Like the squeeze, practicing the zone should be done with light weights—around 5 to 20 pounds. This allows you to manage the weight easily while staying in the tension zone longer and performing more reps. Going too heavy will prevent you from maintaining the zone and getting the full benefit of the exercise.

Remember, don't worry about the weight others are lifting. Focus on your own journey and progress. Everyone starts somewhere, and with patience and consistent practice, you'll reach your goals.

Final Thoughts

The technique of the squeeze and the zone work together to maximize your results. As you practice and refine both, you'll see improvements in both muscle definition and strength. But you need to start humbly, with light weights, and work your way up. Don't rush the process. This is about creating lasting change—physically, mentally, and emotionally.

And most importantly, remember: this journey is for *you*. Your goals, your progress, and your growth are what matter.

CHAPTER 5: WORKOUT SCHEDULE

Before you begin crafting your workout schedule, it's essential to remember that fitness is a lifelong commitment. The psychology of working out emphasizes consistency over short-term goals. You can't approach your fitness journey with a "three months, six months" mindset. As mentioned earlier, consistency is key to success. It doesn't matter what equipment or supplements you have if you're not working out consistently. The routine outlined here is a simple full-body workout, perfect for beginners and advanced athletes alike. It serves as a foundation upon which you can build your personal routine.

Chest

Start with the **Barbell Bench Press** for four sets of six reps. Begin with three sets of lighter weight to warm up, and finish the final set with three controlled reps of a heavier weight close to your maximum. This method, known as the **3:1 West Build** technique, helps with both bulking and shredding. For shredding, use the light-to-heavy approach as described. For bulking, reverse it: start with the heaviest weight you can control for three solid reps, then go lighter for the final set, increasing reps to at least six.

Next, move to the **Barbell Incline Press**, which targets the upper chest. Follow the same **3:1 West Build** technique. Afterward, do the **Barbell Decline Press** to focus on the lower chest.

For a more comprehensive chest workout, include the **Dumbbell Fly** or **Cable Crossover** using the **Zone and Squeeze** method. The **Dumbbell Fly** on a flat bench targets the inner chest, while the **Incline Dumbbell Fly** focuses on the upper chest. To perform the **Cable Crossover** with the Zone and Squeeze method:

- Start with the cables set low. Begin with your hands in front of your thighs and squeeze your chest as your arms come together. Pause at chest level, maintaining the squeeze, then release with control.
- For mid-chest level, your hands should start parallel to your body. Squeeze, pause when your hands are close to each other, then release.
- For the highest cable setting, lean forward and squeeze your chest as you pull your hands almost together in front of you, ensuring you never over-extend your arms.

Lastly, finish your chest routine with the **Dumbbell Pullover**. Use a weight you can control and perform the movement as follows: start with the dumbbells above your chest, elbows slightly bent, then lower the dumbbells behind your head. Squeeze your chest as you bring the dumbbells back to the starting position.

Legs

Leg day requires mental and physical dedication. Begin with the **Squat** using the **3:1 West Build** technique. Lower yourself until your knees are parallel with your butt, then rise, squeezing your glutes at the top of the movement. For your final set, perform a **deep squat**, going lower than usual to target your pelvic area for greater definition.

Next, perform the **Leg Press Machine** and **Calf Press** on the same machine. These exercises are great for overall leg strength and balance. Don't neglect your calves, as they contribute to your overall physique.

For additional leg work, try the **Machine Leg Extension** with the Zone and Squeeze method. Extend your legs until they're almost parallel, stop, then squeeze your thigh muscles before releasing the tension slightly.

Finally, finish with the **Machine Leg Curl** in the prone position, using the 3:1 technique. Squeeze your upper leg muscles and curl your lower legs up, pausing at the peak of the movement before releasing with control.

Arms

The arms are often the most visible part of your physique, making them crucial for aesthetic goals. Start with the **Barbell Curl** using the 3:1 West Build technique, followed by the **Tricep Extension**. Hold the bar overhead and squeeze your triceps before lowering the bar to just above your head. Pause and hold the squeeze before raising it back up.

For alternating exercises, try the **Dumbbell Bicep Curl** and **Dumbbell Tricep Extension**. Both should be performed using the Zone and Squeeze method: squeeze at the peak of each movement and control the release for maximum tension on the muscle.

Next, perform the **Dumbbell Concentration Curl** with your arm resting on your thigh, and alternate with the **Cable One-Arm Tricep Pull-Down**. These exercises are designed to build both strength and definition in your arms.

Back

For the back, begin with the **Cable Seated Row**. Perform two sets with a wide grip and two sets with a close grip. Focus on squeezing your back muscles, and release the tension gradually until the set is complete.

Follow this with the **Barbell Bent-Over Row**, ensuring your back is fully extended during the movement. Finally, do the **Cable Lateral Pulldown**, alternating between wide and close grips for the four sets.

Shoulders

Shoulders are essential for a balanced physique. Start with the **Barbell Shrug**, squeezing your shoulder muscles until your shoulders touch your neck. Hold briefly, then lower with control.

Move on to the **Dumbbell One-Arm Front Raise** and the **Barbell Shoulder Press**, squeezing at the top of each movement. Finish with the **Barbell Upright Row** and **Dumbbell Lateral Raise**, focusing on the squeeze at the top of each rep.

Core

Never skip core exercises, as they are crucial for overall stability. Start with **Weighted Decline Inverted Body Raises**, performing four sets of six reps. Include other core exercises like mountain climbers, flutter kicks, or leg tucks.

Nutrition

Although this book doesn't delve deep into nutrition, a simple approach will go a long way. Aim to burn as much as you consume, and prioritize whole foods like fruits, vegetables, lean meats, and plenty of water. Limit processed foods, sugars, and unhealthy fats. This balanced approach supports a healthy and functional lifestyle.

CONCLUSION

In conclusion, the path to life-changing transformation starts with simple steps, unwavering commitment, and discipline. The Psychology of Working Out begins and ends in the mind. You must mentally prepare yourself and dedicate to a routine that is both worthy and sustainable. Focus, lock in on the results you desire, and commit to the process of achieving those results at the highest level. This book has provided you with the blueprint for success—one that requires no external equipment or gimmicks, just the dedication of your mind and body.

The 3:1 West Build Technique empowers you to build both strength and definition simultaneously, through a variety of movements tailored to your personal fitness journey. The Zone and Squeeze method ensures that every exercise is performed with optimal form and maximum impact. These techniques are not just theories but come from a foundation built on real-world experience—a background of ex-military 13-Fox Fire Support Specialists and over six years of daily gym dedication. They are the result of countless trials and personal growth.
Invest in yourself. The Psychology of Working Out, once mastered, has the potential to transcend fitness, sowing the seeds of discipline and commitment that will extend into every facet of your life. Take a chance on yourself. Take one step closer to becoming the best version of you!

ABOUT THE AUTHOR

Joshua L. D. West

My name is Joshua L. D. West. I have a Bachelor of Science in Psychology. Certified Clinical Mental Health Specialist. Ex-Military and Avid gym enthusiasts. As well as an all-around authentic individual. From Minneapolis, MN. Residing in Northern Italy. All workout techniques and methods are demonstrated visually on TikTok on the channel named @GAWD.BODY444. Search this channel for visual demonstrations and verbal explanations of the exercises and techniques presented in this book. All information in this book is supported by empirically researched data from reputable scholars within their respective fields. You will find resources in the reference section.

* 9 7 9 8 3 0 2 0 0 9 0 0 5 *